ESSENTYIAL GUIDE TO

MOLLOUS

CONTAGIOSUM

Comprehensive Insights and Strategies for Managing Molluscum Contagiosum: An Essential Guide

DR. CASEY LOREN

DISCLAIMER

This book's content is only meant to be used for general informative purposes. Although the author has taken great care to ensure the content is accurate and thorough, no warranties or assurances on the information's accuracy, correctness, or reliability are provided. It is recommended that readers employ their own judgment and discretion when applying any material found in this book to their particular situation.

The information in this book is not intended to replace professional advice, nor is the author an expert in any of the subjects covered. It is recommended that readers consult with experienced professionals regarding any particular issues or concerns.

Any name that may be mentioned or referred in this book does not imply endorsement, recommendation, or relationship on the part of the author with any person, entity, good, website, or association. These references are made only for informational purposes and are not meant to be taken as recommendations or endorsements.

The information contained in this book may cause readers to suffer loss or damage, for which the author disclaims all obligation and accountability. The only people accountable for the decisions and actions taken by readers using the information presented are themselves.

Any names, characters, companies, locations, activities, occasions, and incidents referenced in this book are either made up or the result of the author's imagination. Any likeness to real people, living or dead, or to real things is entirely coincidental.

This book's content may change at any time, without prior notice, according to the author. The onus is on the reader to verify whether there have been any updates or revisions.

The reader accepts the conditions of this disclaimer by reading this book. Please do not read this book or use its contents if you do not agree to these terms.

CHAPTER 1

A BRIEF OVERVIEW OF MOLLUSCUM CONTAGIOSUM

Synopsis and Definition

Molluscum Contagiosum (MC) is a frequent skin infection brought on by the Poxviridae family member molluscum contagiosum virus (MCV). Small, hard, raised lesions on the skin that usually have a center dimple or umbilication are the disease's hallmark. Although these lesions can develop anywhere on the body, the face, trunk, limbs, and genital area are the most frequently affected areas. Since molluscum contagiosum is typically benign and self-limiting, it frequently goes away on its own with time. The illness, however, might last anywhere from a few months to several years.

Molluscum Contagiosum's Past

Molluscum contagiosum has been known about since the early 1800s. Thomas Bateman, a Scottish surgeon, coined the name "molluscum" in 1817. The disease's viral nature was discovered later in the 20th century as improvements in virology and microscopy gave researchers a better understanding of the culprit that caused the illness. Over the years, the disease's understanding has developed, leading to notable advancements in the identification of the virus, its routes of transmission, and the pathology's underlying mechanisms.

Demographics and Epidemiology

Molluscum contagiosum is a disorder that is common around the world and affects people of various ages, ethnicities, and genders. However, sexually active adults, immunocompromised people, and children between the ages of one and ten are the most common populations to experience it. In locations with poor hygiene and high population density, as well as warm, humid conditions, the occurrence rate is higher. Because of the close physical contact, outbreaks can happen among sports teams, schools, and nursery facilities. Males are slightly more likely than females to contract the virus.

Risk factors and causes

Direct skin-to-skin contact, contact with contaminated objects (fomites), or sexual interaction are the three ways that MCV is spread. The following variables raise the chance of developing molluscum contagiosum:

Engaging in contact sports or intimate social interactions might result in close physical touch.

- **Hygiene lapse:** Sharing intimate objects such as garments, towels, or exercise gear.

- **Immune system compromised:** People with diseases including HIV/AIDS, chemotherapy patients, and organ transplant recipients.

- **Atopic dermatitis:** Skin diseases that compromise the skin's barrier function can make viruses easier to enter the body.

Signs and Symptoms

The emergence of tiny, dome-shaped, flesh-colored to pink lesions, usually 2–5 mm in diameter, is the main symptom of molluscum contagiosum. These lesions frequently include a distinctive center dimple. They can be found alone or in groups, and while they usually don't hurt, they occasionally become itchy, red, or inflamed. Picking or scratching the sores increases the risk of developing secondary bacterial infections or autoinoculation—the virus spreading to other skin areas.

Methods of Diagnosis and Testing

Molluscum contagiosum is mostly diagnosed clinically, depending on the distinctive appearance of the lesions. One non-invasive diagnostic technique that can improve central umbilication visualization is dermatoscopy. A skin biopsy could be carried out under unusual circumstances or when the diagnosis is unclear. The diagnosis is confirmed by histopathological testing, which shows characteristic intracytoplasmic inclusion bodies (Henderson-Patterson bodies) within keratinocytes. Testing with the polymerase chain reaction (PCR) can also be used to identify MCV conclusively.

Distinctive Identification

A careful differential diagnosis is necessary because molluscum contagiosum can resemble the appearance of several illnesses. Among them are:

- **Warts:** Warts are often rougher and lack a central umbilication. They are caused by the human papillomavirus (HPV).

- **Folliculitis:** Fibroblast inflammation, commonly seen as papules or pustules.

- **Chickenpox:** Identified by vesicular lesions at different developmental stages.

Basal cell carcinoma: In adults, pearly papules with a central depression may be the presentation.

Effect on Medical Personnel

Despite being benign, molluscum contagiosum can have a major psychological effect, especially on young people. The apparent lesions may result in problems with self-esteem, social stigma, and shame. Genital lesions in adults have the potential to impact romantic relationships and raise worries about STDs. In addition, physical discomfort and the need for medical attention may result from the itching and the possibility of subsequent infections.

Myths and False Beliefs

Molluscum contagiosum is misunderstood about several things, including:

- **Only affects children:** Although prevalent in children, adults are also susceptible to molluscum contagiosum, particularly those who are immunocompromised or engage in sexual activity.

Never needs therapy: Many cases clear up on their own without any help. On the other hand, one can seek treatment to stop the spread or for aesthetic purposes.

- **Very dangerous:** While molluscum contagiosum is usually benign and self-limiting, immunocompromised people may be more susceptible to it.

The Value of Early Identification

Molluscum contagiosum should be detected as soon as possible for several reasons.

Spread Prevention: Prompt detection enables countermeasures against further transmission.

Symptom Management: Early intervention can lessen symptoms and lower the chance of problems such as recurrent bacterial infections.

- **Psychological Benefits:** In children and adolescents in particular, early identification and therapy might lessen the psychological impact.

To ensure better outcomes and lessen the burden of this widespread viral illness, healthcare practitioners and patients alike must have a thorough grasp of molluscum contagiosum, its clinical presentation, and proper therapeutic techniques.

CHAPTER 2

RECOGNIZING THE VIRUS

The Family of Poxviruses

A broad class of DNA viruses recognized for their capacity to infect both vertebrates and invertebrates is referred to as the poxvirus family or Poxviridae. Vaccinia virus, which is utilized in the smallpox vaccine, Molluscum Contagiosum Virus (MCV), and Variola virus (smallpox) are notable members. Poxviruses have an oval or brick-shaped form and are big, complicated, and encapsulated. Unlike many other DNA viruses that replicate in the nucleus, they have the unusual capacity to replicate totally throughout the cytoplasm of the host cell.

Molluscum Contagiosum Virus (MCV) Structure

A big double-stranded DNA virus is called MCV. Its genome, which is roughly 190 kilobase pairs long, encodes for several proteins involved in immune evasion, structural elements, and viral replication. The virus particle, also known as a virion, is a complex structure made up of an outer envelope and a lateral body encircling a core that contains the viral DNA. Surface proteins that are necessary for adhesion and entrance into host cells are used to adorn this envelope.

MCV Genetic Variants

MCV is known to have four genetic variations: MCV-1, MCV-2, MCV-3, and MCV-4. Most infections are caused by MCV-1, which is the most common, especially in youngsters. Adults are more likely to contract MCV-2, which is frequently linked to STDs. These variants differ genetically, which affects their pathogenicity, epidemiology, and potentially even how they interact with the host immune system.

MCV Life Cycle

The MCV life cycle starts when the virus uses endocytosis to enter a host cell. Once within, early gene transcription takes place as the viral core is discharged into the cytoplasm. Following the replication of the viral DNA, intermediate and late gene transcription occurs, resulting in the production of the proteins required for the assembly of new virions. The assembly takes place in cytoplasmic viral factories, and after maturing, the virions are finally discharged to infect other cells through budding or cell lysis.

Modes of Transmission

The main way that MCV is spread is by direct skin-to-skin contact, which includes intercourse. Additionally, it can spread through fomites, which are contaminated toys, clothes, or towels. Autoinoculation is a typical process in which an individual scratches or touches sores on their body, hence spreading the virus to other places of their body. In environments where people are in close physical contact, such as schools, daycare facilities, and sports teams, outbreaks can happen.

Survival in the Environment

Because MCV is comparatively resilient and can linger on surfaces for long periods, contaminated objects can help transmit the virus. Because the virus may survive in damp conditions, places like gym equipment, swimming pools, and shared showers could be possible infection sites. Keeping shared objects clean and practicing good hygiene might help lower the chance of transmission.

Interaction of Pathogen and Host

MCV uses a variety of tactics to subvert the host immune system, enabling infection that lasts a long time. It generates proteins that obstruct interferon signaling pathways, prevent apoptosis (programmed cell death), and reduce inflammation in the host. By using these evasion strategies, the virus can proliferate and propagate without being recognized by the immune system and destroyed.

Reaction Immune to MCV

Both innate and adaptive immunological components are involved in the response to MCV. Through processes like inflammation and the activation of antiviral proteins, the innate immune system first reacts to the viral infection. T cells in particular, which are part of the adaptive immune system, are essential for containing and ultimately eliminating the infection. Nonetheless, MCV can linger for long periods in immunocompromised people, suggesting a complicated interaction between the host's defense mechanisms and viral evasion.

Viral Shedding and Spreadability

MCV particles are highly infectious because they are discharged from infected lesions during viral shedding. Usually, lesions have a core of viral material in the center that is easily disseminated by touch. Shedding can persist for the duration of lesions, emphasizing how crucial it is to cover lesions and maintain proper hygiene to stop transmission.

MCV Laboratory Research

Understanding MCV's biology, pathology, and interactions with the host immune system are the main goals of laboratory study. Research examines how MCV replicates, infects cells, and eludes immune responses using a variety of techniques, such as animal models, cell cultures, and genetic analysis. The objective of these investigations is to pinpoint possible targets for antiviral treatments and enhance methods for avoiding and managing infections.

In conclusion, the Molluscum Contagiosum Virus (MCV) is an important member of the poxvirus family that can infect people due to its special structural and genetic characteristics.

Its contagiousness stems from its capacity to elude the immune system and endure in the environment. To create effective preventative and treatment plans, it is essential to comprehend the life cycle, mechanisms of transmission, and host interactions of the virus.

CHAPTER 3

PRESENTATION OF CLINICAL DATA

Common Skin Illnesses

A viral skin infection known as molluscum contagiosum (MC) is typified by characteristic lesions. Usually, these lesions manifest as:

- **Appearance**: Pearly, flesh-colored papules with a dome form.

Size: Typically have a diameter of 2 to 5 mm.

- **Centre**: They frequently have an umbilication or central dimple.

- **Texture**: Firm, smooth, and occasionally glossy.

Squeezing the central core of these lesions, which contains a white, waxy substance, is one way to express them, however, it is not advised because it could spread the infection.

Frequently Affected Regions

Although MC lesions can develop anywhere on the body, they are most frequently observed on:

- **Youngsters**: Head, neck, and limbs.

- **Adults**: Lower abdomen, inner thighs, and vagina (frequently linked to sexual transmission).

- **Immunocompromised individuals**: More common and may involve unusual locations including the neck and face.

Lesion Development Stages

1. **Incubation**: Before lesions manifest, the virus must incubate for roughly two to seven weeks.

2. **First Lesions**: Firm, flesh-colored papules that are small appear.

3. **Mature Lesions**: These lesions enlarge, umbilicate, and sometimes form a core.

4. **Resolution**: Lesions eventually go away on their own; this normally happens in six to twelve months, though occasionally they take longer.

Differences in Style

- **Gigant Molluscum**: Any lesions more than 15 mm across.

- **Eczematous Molluscum**: Inflamed and itchy skin surrounds the affected area.

Cystic Molluscum: Deep lesions resembling cysts.

- **In individuals with impaired immune systems**: More prevalent, more extensive, and perhaps resistant to therapy.

Adverse Events and Recurrent Infections

- **Bacterial Superinfection**: Pain, swelling, and redness can result from secondary bacterial infections.

- **Scarring**: Picking or scratching lesions might cause scarring.

- **Conjunctivitis**: If the virus penetrates the conjunctiva, lesions close to the eye may result in conjunctivitis.

Distinctions Between Cases in Children and Adults

- **Children**: Usually exhibit facial, torso, and limb lesions. Most of the time, the illness is benign and self-limiting.

Adults: Frequently associated with sexual transmission, genital involvement is more common. Additionally, the inner thighs, lower abdomen, and pubic region may all see an increase in lesions.

Related Skin Illnesses

Common in people with MC, **Eczema** causes irritation and itching around the lesions.

- **Atopic Dermatitis**: People who have this skin condition are more vulnerable to MC.

- **Immunodeficiency-related Conditions**: Lesions that are more severe and pervasive in people who have illnesses like HIV/AIDS.

Psychological Effect

- **Children**: Bullying, social anxiety, and embarrassment can result from visible lesions.

- **Adults**: Sexual relationships and self-esteem may be impacted by genital lesions.

- **General**: Distress and a lower quality of life might result from the stigma attached to visible skin blemishes.

Case Studies and Practical Illustrations

1. A 6-year-old child suffering from atopic dermatitis presents with several MC lesions on their face and arms (Case Study 1). Topical therapy and eczema control are part of the treatment to stop lesion spread.

2. A 30-year-old HIV-positive person presents with extensive and enduring MC lesions in **Case

Study 2**. In addition to cryotherapy for the management of individual lesions, antiretroviral medication aids in the reduction of lesion severity.

3. **Case Study 3**: A sexually active adult, 24 years old, comes with genital and lower abdominal MC lesions. The diagnosis of MC is confirmed, and safe sexual behavior and topical podophyllotoxin are recommended as treatments to stop the spread.

When to Consult a Physician

Lesions classified as **Persistent** occur when they do not go away after a year.

- **Infected or Painful Lesions**: Indications of a secondary infection, such as pus, redness, or warmth.

- **Big or Multiple Lesions**: Especially in people with weakened immune systems.

Cuts Close to the Eyes: May spread to the eye and result in complications such as conjunctivitis.

- **Psychological Distress**: The lesions have a significant emotional or psychological impact.

Seeing a doctor as soon as possible will help with improved symptom management and slow the virus's spread. Topical medications, cryotherapy, and other dermatological treatments are possible forms of treatment.

CHAPTER 4

METHODS OF DIAGNOSIS

Clinical Assessment

The principal technique employed by medical professionals to identify molluscum contagiosum is **Clinical Examination**. An extensive assessment of the skin lesions is part of this examination:

1. **Visual Inspection**: Small, hard, dome-shaped papules with a central umbilication (indentation) are the outward manifestation of Molluscum contagiosum. Lesions often have a diameter of 2 to 5 mm and are flesh-colored, pink, or pearly white.

2. **Location**: Lesions can occur anywhere on the body, however, they are most frequently found on the face, trunk, limbs, and genital areas.

3. **Palpation**: Lesions are typically painless, but if a secondary bacterial infection develops, some may become sensitive or irritating.

4. **Associated Symptoms**: Look for any erythema, inflammation, or secondary infection symptoms that could change how the lesions look.

Skin Examination

Dermatoscopy is a non-invasive diagnostic technique that helps distinguish molluscum contagiosum from other dermatological disorders by magnifying the visibility of skin lesions:

1. **Magnification**: Details about the lesion, like the vascular patterns and central umbilication, are enhanced via dermatoscopy.

2. **Characteristic Findings**: Polylobular white-to-yellow structures and a central punctum are typical dermatoscopic findings of molluscum contagiosum. Blood veins encircle the center core in radial, linear, or dotted patterns.

3. **Advantages**: Dermatoscopy increases the precision of diagnosis and is especially helpful in unusual cases.

Histopathology

In **Histopathology**, tissue samples are examined under a microscope to confirm the diagnosis:

1. **Biopsy Technique**: Usually a punch or shave biopsy is used to remove a tiny sample of skin from a lesion.

2. **Microscopic Features**: Characteristic findings are revealed by histological examination:

- **Epidermal Hyperplasia**: Lobulated growth patterns and thickening of the epidermis.

- **Molluscum Bodies**: Pathognomonic for molluscum contagiosum, are large eosinophilic cytoplasmic inclusions (Henderson-Patterson bodies) within keratinocytes.

3. **Purpose**: When a clinical diagnosis is unclear or lesions are unusual, histopathology can be especially helpful.

Tools for Molecular Diagnostics

By detecting viral DNA, **Molecular Diagnostic Tools** offer accurate identification of the molluscum contagiosum virus (MCV):

1. **PCR-Based Methods**: The most widely used molecular method for identifying MCV DNA is polymerase chain reaction, or PCR.

2. **Sequencing**: MCV can be identified and its subtypes (MCV-1 to MCV-4) can be distinguished using DNA sequencing.

3. **Application**: When other diagnostic techniques prove unsatisfactory, these instruments are employed in difficult patients and research environments.

PCR, or polymerase chain reaction

Viral DNA can be amplified and detected using the extremely sensitive and specific **Polymerase Chain Reaction (PCR)** method:

1. **Sample Collection**: Tissue samples or swabs are taken from lesions.

2. **Procedure**: MCV DNA is amplified in certain portions by PCR, enabling its detection in even minute amounts.

3. **Advantages**: PCR has a high degree of accuracy and can detect MCV even in infections that are early or subclinical.

Laboratory Testing

Serological Tests entail identifying MCV-antibody antibodies in the blood:

1. **Purpose**: The evaluation of past or present infections is the goal of these tests.

2. **Limitations**: Because molluscum contagiosum is a localized infection and other diagnostic techniques are more accurate, serological testing is not frequently utilized in routine clinical practice for molluscum contagiosum diagnosis.

Histopathological analysis

Immunohistochemistry identifies certain antigens in tissue slices using antibodies:

1. **Application**: This method can verify whether MCV proteins are present in tissue samples.

2. **Procedure**: After treating tissue sections with antibodies that are specific to MCV antigens, chromogenic or fluorescent techniques are used to visualize the tissue sections.

3. **Benefit**: In unusual or complex instances, immunohistochemistry might help verify the diagnosis.

Diverse Diagnoses: Disorders Resembling Molluscum

Differential Diagnoses entail separating molluscum contagiosum from other illnesses that appear similarly:

1. **Viral Infections**: Herpes simplex virus infections, warts (caused by HPV).

2. **Bacterial Infections**: impetigo, foliculitis.

3. **Dermatologic Conditions**: milia, basal cell carcinoma, and keratoacanthoma.

4. **Inflammatory Conditions**: acne, eczema.

Diagnostic Difficulties

The following factors may cause **Diagnostic Challenges** in molluscum contagiosum:

1. **Atypical Presentations**: Clinical diagnosis might become more difficult when lesions appear bigger, more frequent, or inflammatory.

2. **Immunocompromised Patients**: People in this category may exhibit widespread, enduring, or unusual lesions.

3. **Secondary Infections**: Bacterial superinfection can change how lesions look, which complicates diagnosis.

Molluscum contagiosum is becoming more and more manageable with the use of **telemedicine**:

1. **Remote Consultations**: Patients can obtain specialist care more easily by having video consultations for dermatologic exams.

2. **Image Sharing**: To facilitate remote diagnosis, high-resolution pictures of lesions can be shared with medical professionals.

3. **Follow-Up Care**: Telemedicine enables continued treatment progress monitoring and problem management.

4. **Advantages**: Better simplicity of use, accessibility, and capacity to handle situations in isolated locations or during public health emergencies.

To guarantee that medical professionals are equipped with the necessary knowledge to properly diagnose and treat molluscum contagiosum, this book offers a thorough review of the various diagnostic procedures.

CHAPTER 5

OPTIONS FOR TREATMENT

Vigilant Awaiting and Instinctive Settlement

Watchful waiting is keeping an eye on the situation without taking any quick action. Lesions caused by Molluscum contagiosum usually go away on their own in six to twelve months. To stop the lesions from spreading or developing into secondary infections, patients should refrain from picking or scratching during this time. Patients should be informed about the disease's natural progression and reassured that treatment is typically not necessary.

Methods of Physical Removal

1. **Cryotherapy:** Liquid nitrogen is used to freeze the lesions. Although it's a popular and

useful technique, it could irritate skin temporarily and create discomfort.

2. **Curettage:** A medical practitioner removes the lesions with a sharp tool known as a curette. Although it's short, it can need local anesthesia and leave some tiny scars.

3. **Laser Therapy:** Using concentrated light energy, laser treatment locates and eliminates the lesions. Although it can result in short-term redness and swelling, it is accurate and frequently used for bigger or resistant lesions.

4. **Needling:** To release the virus's contents, this method entails puncturing the lesions with a needle. Because of the possibility of virus propagation and scarring, it is not as widely used.

Topical Interventions

1. **Imiquimod:** Induces an immunological reaction against the virus by stimulating the skin's immune system. It is put directly onto the lesions and as a side effect, skin discomfort may occur.

2. **Podophyllotoxin:** An additional topical treatment for the lesions is also an option. It functions by interfering with the process of viral replication. Owing to its toxicity, it should be used carefully and under medical supervision.

3. **Retinoids:** Topically administered, these derivatives of vitamin A can shorten the duration and size of lesions. By encouraging skin cell turnover, they function.

4. Cannabidin is a topical blistering agent that causes the lesions to blister and eventually fall off. Due to its potency, it is usually used in a healthcare context.

Systemic Interventions

Systemic treatments, which may involve oral antiviral drugs or immunomodulators, are often saved for severe cases or people with impaired immune systems. Because of the possible interactions and adverse effects, these treatments need to be closely monitored by a medical practitioner.

Natural Therapies and At-Home Remedies

Although molluscum contagiosum is treated with a variety of natural therapies and home remedies, its effectiveness is frequently questionable. These could include several herbal medicines, apple cider vinegar, and tea tree oil. It's imperative to use caution when attempting these and to speak with a healthcare professional first.

Handling Difficulties

Secondary bacterial infections are an uncommon but possible consequence of molluscum contagiosum, particularly if lesions are touched or inflamed. Complications can be avoided by practicing good hygiene, not sharing personal objects, and maintaining dry, clean skin.

Immunocompromised Patients' Treatment

Molluscum contagiosum instances can be more severe or persistent in immunocompromised people, such as those on immunosuppressive medication or living with HIV. In these situations, treatment may involve systemic and topical medications in addition to careful observation for side effects.

Treatment Costs and Accessibility

Depending on several variables, including geography, insurance coverage, and the particular treatment selected, the cost and accessibility of therapies might differ significantly. While some treatments, like laser therapy or some topical drugs, may be more expensive and require medical skill, others, including watchful waiting and simple hygiene practices, are more accessible and cost-effective.

To sum up, there are a variety of therapy choices for molluscum contagiosum, including topical medications, systemic therapies, home cures, and other physical removal techniques in addition to cautious waiting. The severity of the ailment, patient preferences, cost, and accessibility all play a role in the treatment decision. Medical professionals must inform patients of their options and customize treatment regimens to meet their unique requirements.

CHAPTER 6

PREVENTIVE TECHNIQUES

Principles of Personal Hygiene

Hand washing with soap and water regularly can aid in halting the spread of molluscum contagiosum.

Steer clear of exchanging personal goods like clothes, razors, or towels to reduce the chance of infection.

Avoiding Direct Contact with Skin

- To lessen the risk of catching the virus, advise people to stay away from places that are directly in contact with their skin.

If it is not possible to prevent direct contact, cover lesions with clothing or bandages as a barrier.

Safe Utilisation of Public Spaces

Encourage people to use caution when they are in public spaces like gyms or swimming pools, as shared equipment or contact with contaminated surfaces can readily spread the virus.

Promote the usage of sanitized surfaces and the use of personal towels.

Safeguarding Members of the Home

Inform family members about the virus and how to stop it from spreading to other members of the home.

Encourage infected people to use separate bedding, clothes, and towels to reduce contact with family members who are not afflicted.

Vaccination's Role

- Talk about the possible contribution of vaccination to the prevention of molluscum contagiosum, despite the absence of a specialized vaccine at this time.

- Stay informed about any advancements in the development of this virus's vaccine.

Programmes for Community Awareness

- Encourage neighborhood campaigns that increase knowledge of molluscum contagiosum, how it spreads, and how to prevent it.

- Offer community members educational resources and materials.

Initiatives for Education in Schools

- Work along with educational institutions to develop educational initiatives regarding skin illnesses, such as molluscum contagiosum.

Stress the value of pupils maintaining good personal hygiene and avoiding skin-to-skin contact.

Professional Safety

In environments where there is frequent close contact, such as healthcare settings, stress the importance of wearing personal protection equipment (PPE) and following good hygiene procedures.

Inform staff members about the symptoms and indicators of molluscum contagiosum to encourage early detection and prevention.

Keeping Sports from Transmitting

Urge athletes to follow proper hygiene practices, like taking a shower after a sporting event and not sharing towels or equipment.

- To reduce the spread of illnesses during training and contests, think about establishing policies for athletes who are currently infected.

- Warn tourists that they can come into contact with Molluscum contagiosum in crowded or shared areas when traveling.

When traveling, bring supplies for personal hygiene and take precautions against potential hazards.

A culture of awareness and proactive actions, along with a complete approach to prevention, can greatly lower the risk of molluscum contagiosum transmission in a variety of contexts.

CHAPTER 7

HAVING MOLLUSCUM CONTAGIOSUM IN YOUR HOME

Daily Routine for Skincare

When using Molluscum contagiosum in your everyday skincare regimen, you should concentrate on mild washing and moisturizing. Don't scrub too hard as this could aggravate the sores; instead, use gentle soap. To keep the skin hydrated, pat the afflicted areas dry and then apply a calming moisturizer.

Managing Itching and Unease

Molluscum contagiosum frequently causes itching and pain. Calamine lotion or over-the-counter anti-itch lotions can be used to treat these symptoms. To stop the virus from spreading or leading to other infections, refrain from scratching.

Handling the Psychological and Emotional Effects

Emotionally taxing living with molluscum contagiosum can be particularly difficult for kids and teenagers. It's critical to have honest conversations about the illness, ask for medical professionals' assistance, and, if necessary, think about counseling or therapy.

Support Teams and Guidance

Getting counseling or joining support groups can be beneficial for coping mechanisms and emotional support. These resources can assist you in overcoming the difficulties associated with having molluscum contagiosum and in making connections with people who share your experiences.

Kids and Attendance at School

It's critical to discuss molluscum contagiosum in youngsters with teachers and school officials. Inform them of the virus's minimal transmission risk and stress the need to maintain good hygiene to stop it from spreading.

Handling Social Shame

Regrettably, misconceptions regarding the molluscum contagiosum's mode of spread can lead to societal stigma. Inform people about the virus, stress that it is safe, and encourage compassion and understanding.

Interaction with Friends and Family

Having frank conversations with loved ones and friends is essential to getting assistance and lowering anxiety related to the illness. Answer their inquiries and provide accurate facts on molluscum contagiosum.

Extended Skincare

Maintaining healthy skin once the molluscum contagiosum lesions have healed requires consistent application of good skincare practices. To avoid sun damage, wear sunscreen, and moisturize frequently to avoid drying out.

Keeping an eye out for repeats

Molluscum contagiosum usually goes away on its own, however it might reoccur. Continue to be on the lookout for any new lesions on your skin. Should you observe any changes or have any concerns, speak with your healthcare physician.

Remaining Up to Date and Informed

Consult trustworthy sources, like medical journals, respected websites, and healthcare specialists, to stay informed about molluscum contagiosum. Stay informed about any new advancements or available treatment alternatives.

You may effectively manage molluscum contagiosum and reduce its impact on your everyday life and well-being by adhering to these instructions and being educated.

CHAPTER 8

PARTICULAR POPULATIONS OF MOLLUSCUM CONTAGIOSUM

Attention to Paediatrics

Children frequently get molluscum contagiosum, especially those who are between the ages of one and ten. Because of the intimate contact that occurs in playgroups, daycare centers, and schools, it spreads easily among youngsters. Small, painless, raised lesions on the skin, usually on the hands, arms, and face, are a common feature of pediatric cases. Children may need to be treated gently because of their sensitive skin and the chance of scarring. While topical therapies and cryotherapy are frequently employed, great care is taken to reduce young patients' discomfort and psychological effects.

Sexual Transmission and Adults:

Although it is more common in children, adults can still have Molluscum Contagiosum, particularly if they have compromised immune systems or participate in activities that encourage skin-to-skin contact. Intimate contact has the potential to transmit sexually and cause genital lesions. Adult Molluscum management frequently entails treating the psychological effects, since genital sores can be extremely distressing. Topical therapies or in-office procedures may be used as treatment methods in conjunction with prevention and safe sexual practice education.

People with Compromised Immunities

People with weakened immune systems—those living with HIV/AIDS or receiving immunosuppressive treatment, for example—are more vulnerable to serious and widespread Molluscum Contagiosum infections. Because of the possibility of rapid lesion spread and durability, these instances may need more intensive treatment strategies and vigilant monitoring. Immunologists, dermatologists, and infectious disease specialists are frequently involved in the interdisciplinary management of Molluscum in immunocompromised patients to customize treatment to meet each patient's specific medical requirements.

Sports Fans and Athletes

The close quarters in training facilities or locker rooms, coupled with skin-to-skin contact, can put athletes and sports enthusiasts—especially those participating in contact sports or activities involving shared equipment—at higher risk of contracting Molluscum Contagiosum. To reduce the danger of spread among sporting communities, preventive measures like good hygiene, not sharing personal things, and quick treatment of any suspicious lesions are crucial.

Due to a weakened skin barrier, patients with atopic dermatitis, a chronic inflammatory skin disorder, may be more vulnerable to Molluscum Contagiosum. Eczema lesions can act as ports of entry for the virus, resulting in infections with Molluscum that are more widespread and long-lasting. When treating Molluscum in people with atopic dermatitis, it's common to treat the two disorders at the same time, emphasizing targeted antiviral treatments, skin barrier restoration, and inflammation management.

Women Who Are Expecting

Pregnant women with molluscum contagiosum need to take extra precautions because there is a chance that the fetus could be exposed during birthing. Although the virus does not usually inflict significant damage on the unborn child, steps can be taken to reduce the possibility of transfer during childbirth. There aren't many alternatives for treatment during pregnancy; the main strategies are conservative ones and close observation to make sure the virus doesn't interfere with the pregnancy or birth process.

Senior Citizens

Even though Molluscum Contagiosum is more frequently observed in young people and children, it can also afflict elderly patients, particularly those residing in close quarters in assisted living or nursing homes. A customized approach to management may be necessary for older persons due to their comorbidities, fragile skin, and possible medication interactions. Dermatologists and geriatric specialists frequently work together to maximize treatment results while attending to any underlying medical issues.

Disabled Individuals

Managing Molluscum Contagiosum can provide particular obstacles for people with disabilities, such as trouble identifying and expressing symptoms, getting access to medical care, and following treatment plans. Support from carers and medical professionals is essential in helping these people, as they provide information, help with cleanliness, and the right medications to manage the infection and enhance quality of life.

Medical Professionals

In their professional contexts, healthcare professionals—especially those in the fields of infectious diseases, dermatology, and pediatrics—may come into contact with Molluscum Contagiosum. Strict attention to infection control procedures is necessary to avoid occupational exposure and transmission among healthcare workers and patients. These procedures include hand cleanliness, the use of personal protective equipment (PPE), and the safe disposal of contaminated objects.

Special Population Case Studies

Case studies about certain populations offer significant insights into the clinical manifestation, obstacles, and approaches to managing

Molluscum contagiosum. These instances demonstrate the value of tailored treatment, interdisciplinary teamwork, and continuous research to enhance results and maximize patient care for a range of patient populations.

To personalize treatment strategies and ensure optimal results for patients across the lifespan, addressing Molluscum Contagiosum in particular populations necessitates a comprehensive approach that takes into account characteristics such as age, immunological state, underlying medical disorders, and unique risk factors.

CHAPTER 9

FUTURE PROSPECTS FOR RESEARCH

Present Research Patterns

The following areas are the focus of current molluscum contagiosum (MC) research:

- **Genomic Analysis:** To comprehend the genetic composition of the virus and how it changes over time, researchers are utilizing cutting-edge genomic tools.

- **Immunological Response:** To create more effective treatment plans, there is an increasing interest in researching the innate and adaptive immunological responses to MC.

Epidemiological Studies: Investigations into the incidence of MC in various demographic groups and geographical areas, as well as risk factors for infection and the dynamics of transmission, are still underway.

Novel therapeutic strategies for the treatment of MC have surfaced in recent years:

- **Topical Immunomodulators:** To enhance the immune response against MC lesions, some research has investigated the use of topical immunomodulators such as imiquimod.

- **Photodynamic Therapy:** This targets and eliminates MC lesions by combining photosensitizing drugs with light-based therapy.

- **Antiviral medicines:** Scholars are examining the effectiveness of topical and systemic antiviral medicines in managing multicommunicative infections (MC outbreaks).

The following are being done to create a vaccination against MC:

- **Subunit vaccinations:** To elicit protective immunity, researchers are investigating the use of subunit vaccinations that target particular MC virus proteins.

- **DNA vaccinations:** By inducing an immune response to viral components, DNA-based vaccinations are also being investigated as a potential preventive measure against MC infection.

Progress in Diagnostic Methods

The precision and speed of MC diagnosis have increased due to advancements in diagnostic techniques:

PCR-Based Tests: Clinical samples containing MC virus DNA can be detected with excellent sensitivity and specificity using polymerase chain reaction (PCR) assays.

- **Immunohistochemistry:** Skin biopsy specimens stained with immunohistochemical staining can be used to confirm the presence of the MC virus in lesions.

Point-of-Care Tests: Quick and simple diagnostic tools are being created to help identify the MC virus in clinical settings.

Comprehending Viral Pathophysiology

The goal of research is to understand the pathophysiology of MC:

- **Viral Entry and Replication:** Research focuses on how the MC virus moves throughout the skin, replicates, and gains entry into host cells.

- **Immune Evasion:** Scientists are looking at how the virus sidesteps human defenses and causes enduring infections.

Lesion Development: Targeted therapy development is aided by an understanding of the molecular mechanisms underlying lesion formation.

MCV Genetic Research

The MC virus's (MCV) genetic research is illuminating the diversity and evolution of the virus:

- **Genomic Sequencing:** Complete genome sequencing of MCV strains from various geographical locations sheds light on the genetic diversity and diversity of the virus.

- **Mutational Analysis:** Researching changes in viral genes aids in the understanding of antiviral resistance and the identification of possible therapeutic targets.

- **Phylogenetic Studies:** Using phylogenetic analysis, epidemiological research can be aided in tracing the emergence and dissemination of MCV strains.

Longitudinal Research on the Development of Disease

Studies that follow a subject's course across time to monitor MC infection

- **Natural History:** These studies show how MC lesions naturally develop, including rates of spontaneous remission and recurrence.

Outcomes of Treatment: Extended patient monitoring during treatment aids in evaluating the efficacy of different therapy approaches.

Impact on Quality of Life: Researchers assess the psychological effects of MC on patients, particularly youngsters, as well as the variables affecting the severity of the illness.

Implications for Public Health

MC has important consequences for public health:

- **Transmission Dynamics:** Putting preventive measures in place requires an understanding of how MC spreads throughout communities and healthcare settings.

Outbreak Management: Guidelines for handling communicable diseases (MC) outbreaks, such as case identification, isolation, and contact tracing, are developed by public health agencies.

- **Health Education:** Initiatives to raise public awareness inform people about the spread of MC, preventative measures, and getting medical attention.

Upcoming Difficulties in Prevention and Treatment

There are numerous obstacles to overcome in the prevention and treatment of MC:

- **Antiviral Resistance:** Prolonged use of some medications may cause resistance development, hence it is important to monitor for antiviral resistance.

- **Vaccination Obstacles:** Overcoming technological and immunological obstacles is necessary to develop a vaccination against MC that is both safe and effective.

Global Access: It is still difficult to guarantee fair access to MC diagnosis, treatments, and immunizations, especially in areas with few resources.

Global Health Organisations' Contributions

International health organizations are essential to the fight against MC:

- **Research Funding:** Institutions provide funding for studies that try to advance MC prevention, diagnosis, and treatment methods.

- **Guideline Development:** They work with specialists to create evidence-based guidelines for managing mental illness (MC) on a national and worldwide scale.

- **Capacity Building:** Initiatives related to global health assist in developing capacity in fields including epidemiology, public health surveillance, and laboratory diagnostics for MC.

The understanding and treatment of molluscum contagiosum are improving thanks to these study fields and ongoing difficulties, which is good news for patients and public health initiatives around the world.

CHAPTER 10

MATERIALS AND ASSISTANCE

Portals for Online Information

Comprehensive information on molluscum contagiosum can be found on websites such as WebMD, Mayo Clinic, and the American Academy of Dermatology. They go over every topic imaginable, including preventative techniques, treatment alternatives, and symptoms. These portals are trustworthy resources for anyone looking for thorough and current information regarding the illness.

Advocacy Groups for Patients

Patients suffering from molluscum contagiosum may find great assistance from associations such as the American Academy of Dermatology Association and the National Eczema Association.

They offer guidance, educational resources, and occasionally even treatment funding. These organizations frequently provide online forums where sufferers can interact with others going through comparable difficulties.

Associations for Professional Medicine

Two important professional bodies that offer guidelines and resources to medical practitioners treating molluscum contagiosum are the American Academy of Dermatology and the American Academy of Paediatrics. They provide training opportunities, instructional materials, and updates on the most effective methods for diagnosis and treatment.

Governmental Health Organisations

Reliable sources of information on molluscum contagiosum are government organizations such as the National Institutes of Health (NIH) and the Centres for Disease Control and Prevention

(CDC). They provide advice on the illness's management, prevention, and public health initiatives.

Research Studies and Clinical Trials

Research studies and clinical trials are essential for expanding our knowledge of molluscum contagiosum and creating novel treatment approaches. Patients who wish to take part in clinical trials can obtain information by visiting websites such as ClinicalTrials.gov, which provides a list of current studies and qualifying requirements.

Brochures and Educational Materials

Brochures and other teaching materials about molluscum contagiosum are frequently produced by government organizations, patient advocacy groups, and healthcare providers. These sites address issues including signs and symptoms, modes of transmission, available treatments, and preventative measures. Both people and healthcare providers can benefit from them.

Smartphone Apps for Skincare

Information about molluscum contagiosum may be included in some smartphone apps that concentrate on skin health. Applications such as DermNet NZ and VisualDx provide instructional information and visual aids for a range of skin disorders, including molluscum contagiosum.

Services for Telehealth

Patients can conveniently visit healthcare specialists remotely regarding molluscum contagiosum with the help of telehealth services. Virtual visits with dermatologists and other specialists who can diagnose and suggest treatment for the illness are available through platforms such as Teladoc, Amwell, and Doctor On Demand.

Programmes for Community Health

Programs centered on skin health and infectious disorders like molluscum contagiosum may be offered by neighborhood associations and health authorities in your area. Screenings, instructional seminars, and resources for treatment and prevention are a few examples of these programs.

Support Services Contact Details

People can get in touch with government health authorities, patient advocacy groups, and healthcare providers directly for support and assistance with molluscum contagiosum. These services frequently have contact information on their websites, helplines, and support forums.

Through the utilization of these resources and support services, people who are impacted by molluscum contagiosum can obtain important information, establish connections with other individuals for assistance, and obtain help on properly managing the condition.